# The Little Book of
# DETOX

## JANE SCRIVNER

PIATKUS

First published in 1999 by
Judy Piatkus (Publishers) Ltd
5 Windmill Street
London W1P 1HF
www.piatkus.co.uk

Reprinted 1999, 2000

**The moral right of the author has been asserted**

*A catalogue record for this book is available
from the British Library*

ISBN 0-7499-1994-9

Designed by Zena Flax
Typeset by Phoenix Photosetting, Chatham, Kent
Printed and bound in Great Britain by
Redwood Books, Trowbridge, Wilts

*To Kevin for suggesting it,
Rachel for reacting so quickly
and me for getting it done.*

# About the author

Jane Scrivner established The British School of Complementary Therapy in Harley Street in 1991. It offers full and part-time courses in a range of therapies including therapeutic massage, reflexology and aromatherapy. One of the most popular treatments at the clinic is the detox and anti-cellulite programme.

Jane Scrivner lives in Stratford-upon-Avon and London, and her previous books include *Detox Your Mind* and the bestselling *Detox Yourself* (both Piatkus).

# How to use this book

Carry it with you always and when you feel 'toxed' – stressed, tired, lethargic, in need of cheering up, sluggish, in need of a boost, or fuzzy headed –

Simply open the book,
pick a page,
and do it!

Everything is designed to make you feel good – physically, emotionally and mentally.

*Give it a try – you have nothing to lose and everything to gain.*
*You deserve it!*

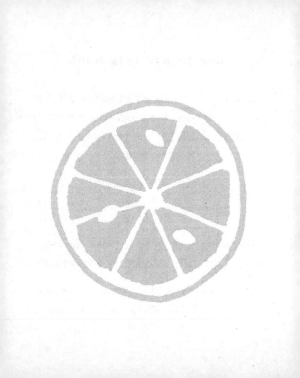

# Water, water, water

Drink 3 pints or 1.5 litres of filtered or bottled water every day.

It rehydrates, revitalises, cleans your skin, flushes you out and invigorates.

## Junk the caffeine

Reduce tea and coffee to one cup per day
for a whole month and then cut out
caffeine altogether.

See how your skin tone changes,
your sleep gets deeper and you feel
more relaxed.

# Wake up call

Turn the shower to cold for 30 seconds every morning.

A cold shower leaves you feeling warm, invigorated and awake.

## Make with the veggies

Eat at least 5 servings of fresh vegetables
every day –

and make sure 3 of them are *raw*:
raw food is raw energy!

# Eat brain foods

Stimulate and nourish your mind
by eating food for thought.

Choline in vegetables and eggs –
aids memory.
DMAE in fish especially anchovies and
sardines – improves memory and
increases intelligence.
Inositol in grapefruit and cabbage –
nourishes brain cells.
Niacin in liver, kidney, fish, eggs, poultry,
avocado and peaches – creates a healthy
nervous system and better brain function.
Carbohydrates in pulses, rice, potatoes –
provides essential energy for our brains
and central nervous system.

# Refresh at the gym

If you have a gym membership and don't use it then just get down there.

Would you pay £500 for a swim?
£460 for a sauna?
£100 for a workout?

No? Well, if you don't use the facilities very much you have probably already done so. Use what you already have and get value for money and fitness for life.

# Fruity, fruity

Eat at least 3 servings of fresh fruit per day
– a serving is a whole fruit or a slice the
size of a tablespoon.

Give yourself a revitalising energy boost.

## Change a negative
## to a positive

If something bad happens think of 4 steps
to turn it into something good.

You miss your bus;
You have 20 minutes to nip and buy
some groceries;
You call a friend and invite them for supper;
You have a pleasant impromptu evening.

Decontaminate your mind. Negative to
positive – so easy when you know how.

# Try some freshly sprouted beans or seeds

Freshly sprouted beans and seeds have a massive nutrient content which is easy to digest. There are many to try – including cress, chick peas, lentils, mustard, oats and sunflower seeds.

Flavour, colour and texture with ultimate nutrition.

Sprinkle them on a salad or pack them into a sandwich and crunch away.

## Learn 4 new things

Shake up your brain cells and learn
4 new things today.

Your PIN number.
That rhyme about the length of days
in the month.
A new joke to tell.
Open a dictionary and learn a new word.

# Develop a dressing

Take fresh oils, fresh herbs and some fruits
and blend yourself a fantastically fragrant
new dressing, packed with flavour
and nutrients.

Lettuce takes on a whole new meaning
in a new outfit.

# Nature's little helper

Garlic wards off germs, boosts your
immune system and increases circulation –
take an odourless tablet a day and never
catch a cold again.

# Juice up your life

Juicing gives you all the nutrients you need in a glass with no chomping, peeling or chewing.

Choose your favourite fruits and juice them – either individually or in energy-boosting combinations.

Try and achieve a colourful effect by juicing each fruit individually and pouring slowly in to the glass in rotation – a rainbow elixir for life.

# Take a risk

Challenge your comfort zone and see how brilliant you feel once you have achieved something you never dreamed possible.

Take a parachute jump.
Touch a snake or spider.
Sing some karaoke in a public bar.
Do a bungee jump.

Yikes! You see, you can do anything if you try.

# Take a liver tonic every day

We wash our hair and our faces every day
but we cannot take out our internal organs
and rinse them through, so give your liver
a boost today.

Eat a bunch of red grapes.
Take a fresh garlic clove or odourless
garlic tablet.
Drink a glass of carrot or beetroot juice
every day.
Drink some dandelion or fennel tea.

# Get into visualisations

If there is something that is worrying you or playing on your mind then try visualisation. Simply get into a relaxed position and visualise yourself in the situation with everything turning out for the best. Then when the event actually happens you will know exactly what to do to make things turn out fine and dandy.

# Do something you have never done before

It is very easy to stop trying new things –
we feel too old or not ready for change or
cannot be bothered. Well, try something
new and see how it changes you for the best.

Go to the theatre.
Eat snails.
Make a cake.
Draw a picture.
Jump in a puddle.

Have a go – and teach the old dog
a new trick!

## Eucalyptus – disinfectant of the natural world

Burning Eucalyptus oil in a burner or sniffing it from a handkerchief is reported to kill off 70 per cent of all airborne germs.

When there is a bug going round or everyone has a cold, get the Eucalyptus bubbling and drive the germs away.

Keep yourself germ free and fighting fit.

# Yell loudly, expand your lungs and banish stress

You know how when you feel tense or stressed you just want to shout or hit something – or someone!?

So do it. Go out into the countryside, down to the beach or just make sure the neighbours are out and yell and scream, stamp your feet and gnash your teeth.

Feels great doesn't it? It does you good as well – and it stops you thumping anyone.

# Convenience Foods?

Full of fats, toxins, preservatives,
E numbers, colourings, sugars, processed
foods and flours.

Low in vitamins, minerals, nutrients,
freshness and energy.

How convenient is that?

# Rosemary

Use Rosemary essential oil as a
balancer of moods.

Burn it, use it in self massage or bathe in it.

Inhale deeply and bring yourself
back together.

# Paint a picture

Or draw one. Just get out the paints or pencils and doodle away. You are not looking for a masterpiece, just something that opens up the creative part of your mind.

Blow away the cobwebs – get creative!

# Mandarin, Ylang Ylang or Rose

... are all oils used for boosting self-worth. Unfortunately Rose is incredibly expensive so sink into a bath with a few drops of Ylang Ylang or Mandarin in some base oil and emerge when you rule the world!

# Lemongrass

Another oil to use at home, Lemongrass is refreshing, cleansing and spicy. It stimulates digestion and eases a nervous stomach.

It also promotes the removal of toxins from the body and is both antiseptic and bactericidal – need any more reasons to get some!?

# Detox your wardrobe

Go through your old clothes and take all the ones you don't wear to a charity shop.

The staff are really grateful for the free stock;
so are all the customers that buy it;
and so are all the people that benefit from the charity funds generated.

# Flush out fluids

Drink Dandelion tea on a daily basis and flush out the excess fluids in your body.

Alternatively put Dandelion leaves in your salads and crunch your way to the same benefits.

## Feng Shui

Have your whole house feng shui'd and detox your living space of anything negative. The cost will almost certainly be recovered when the feng shui specialist discovers how you can capitalise on your wealth area.

For a budget version seek out your local course and see if the students need 'project fodder'.

# Don't eat red meat

Give your digestive system a holiday and
cut out red meat for a whole month.

Feel the benefits and then
cut it out altogether.

# Nothing but a dreamer ...

Allow yourself dream time.

Imagine yourself carried away in your imagination, detox negative thoughts and enjoy the possibility of anything happening.

Return to this world refreshed and renewed – and remember, if you don't have dreams then they can't come true!

# Turn off the TV

Turn off the TV and do something else.

Have a conversation.
Get a job done that you have avoided so far.
Phone a friend.
Take a relaxing bath.
Listen to music.
Listen to the radio.

Do anything to make a change.

# Laughter

Do something to make yourself laugh.
Laughter is one of the best stress relievers
and relaxers.

See a funny film.
Read a funny book.
Get friends round for a good old giggle.
See a comedy show.

# Meditate

Meditation relaxes the mind and leaves it receptive to new things and fresh approaches.

Sit comfortably, totally supported by cushions, blankets, chairs etc.
Close your eyes and focus on your breathing.
Take your mind through your body and watch your breath relax each and every limb.
Start at your feet and when the breath reaches the top of your head, bring your breath back into the room, open your eyes and get on with your day – cool and calm.

# Don't just go through the process

Processed foods contain lots of things that we waste our time eating as we cannot use them for nutrition, so save time in your life and eliminate processed foods.
Feel great knowing that everything that goes in is pure fuel for life.

# Do a mini, mini fast

Eat your last meal before 6.00 p.m. and then leave breakfast until after 9.00 a.m. and give your digestive system a full 15 hours to totally clean out and process all residual foods in the body.

Make the meals either side of your mini, mini fast consist of fresh fruit and vegetables and enhance your fast even further.

Cleanse your body and boost your immune system.

# Apply the 6 month rule

Clear out your room and bag up all the things you don't use but cannot bear to throw away. Put the bag away in a cupboard or cellar and if you haven't needed any of it for 6 months then you really don't need it. Donate the contents to someone who could really benefit from actually using them.

# Get to know your herbal teas

Herbs can boost you, relax you, invigorate and much much more. Choose a new herbal tea each week and find yourself a favourite.

# Take a kidney tonic every day

Take a spoonful of honey in a cup
of hot water;
drink a glass of cranberry juice;
or eat half a medium melon.

Give your kidneys a boost and
feel the benefits.

## Play

Go out and play – completely
unadulterated fun and nonsense.

It doesn't have to mean anything.
It doesn't have to be a means to an end.
It doesn't have to involve anyone else.
It should be your own playtime.

Then go back inside and get on with your
day – happy and uplifted.

# Eat oily fish

Rollmops, kippers, salmon, sardines and mackerel are all high in Omega-3 fatty acids. Research has shown that these can:

discourage heart disease;
help to reduce the risk of cancer;
give you a glowing skin;
help with arthritis.

Need I say more?

# Fix something

Remember that shirt that has a missing button? Well, sew the button on today so that next time you need the shirt you can actually wear it.

Fix something that needs a small repair and make a big difference.

# Try organic

Try to eat entirely organic food for a week.

Taste the new flavours and feel the extra crunch as you bite into foods that are jam-packed with twice the goodness and none of the badness.

# Clean out your food cupboards

Revitalise your food cupboards by throwing out everything that has passed its sell-by date.

You will most likely gain a whole free shelf just by getting rid of foods you couldn't eat anyway!

## Moisturise your skin every day

Get glowing skin by putting moisture back.

Drink water.
Use natural oils to moisturise.
Eat fruits high in water content –
grapes, pineapple, plums.
Spritz your face with ice cold filtered water
to give a splash of energy and tone.

## Do 30 minutes of exercise every other day

Climb the stairs.
Walk to work.
Walk to the shops.
Work out.
Vacuum every room.

This will keep you fit and healthy, get rid of
the extra pounds and bulges and make you
feel energised.

### Reduce sugar

Don't add sugar to anything. If you need sweetness then add a small amount of natural honey to help you phase it out and eventually cut out sugars altogether.

Eating less sugar allows you more calorie space to eat more fruit, vegetables, rice and grains – foods high in fibre, vitamins, minerals and energy.

### Sit up straight!

Don't slump. Give your internal o[...] room to spread and operate i[...] optimum space they need and d[...] Your body will be able to detox e[...] leaving you feeling healthy and re[...]

# Breathe!

Relax your stomach muscles;
Breathe in through your nose for
the count of 4;
Take the air to your belly and hold for 4;
Breathe out through your mouth for
the count of 8.

Give your body time to fully benefit from
the breath of life.

# The great eliminator

Locate the acupressure point called 'The great eliminator' – found in the fleshy bit between the thumb and forefinger – and hold it with the thumb and forefinger from the other hand. Push in and squeeze slowly and firmly. It may feel tender, so hold and release until the tenderness goes.

The great eliminator is brilliant in times of stress, tension or just the common or garden headache.

# Spend a day with no spending

Close your purse or wallet at 6.00 p.m. and don't open it until 6.00 a.m. 36 hours later.

See just how much fun you can have and imagination you can use by spending nothing – you can earn but you can't spend.

Hold a car boot sale.
Tidy out the house.
Watch all your home videos.
Visit friends you haven't seen in ages.
Eat all the food in the house that is about to go off.

# Give up smoking now

It's bad for you and you know it. It reduces
your life expectancy and it may even
reduce the life expectancy of others
around you.

Give it up, don't do it anymore, stop it!
There is no excuse.

Eliminate harmful toxins from your life and
get your body back in balance.

# Lose weight instantly

Check your key ring. Do you use all the keys still? If not, get rid of them. You don't need to carry the excess weight around every day.

# Massage

Have a massage once a month. Pay for one
or do it yourself – there are plenty of
practitioners and books on self massage in
the shops. Massage helps eliminate toxins
so once a month you are truly detoxing.

# Evening Primrose oil

Taking Evening Primrose oil will help to reduce stress and balance your hormones. Stay calm and balanced with just one a day.

# Go natural

Try to stop taking painkillers.
If you get a headache use lavender oil.
If you are tense then stretch and shrug
your muscles.
For stomach cramps try deep breathing
and camomile in a gentle abdomen
massage.

Try natural remedies in favour of reaching
for the painkillers.

# Take time to smell the roses

If you are busy or preoccupied then make
sure you take time to 'smell the roses'.

Look at the scenery when riding into work.
Stop and smell some flowers instead of
just seeing how they look.
Walk around your garden to see
what's growing.

It doesn't take long but it's just brilliant for
putting things into perspective.

# Give up on salt

Salt is crucial to survival but we can generally get all the salt we need by following a balanced diet.

Stop adding salt and avoid anything in brine solutions, with sodium added as an ingredient or any salted foods.

Once your taste buds get the chance to do their job you will find that foods do have some wonderful flavours of their own.

# Zap the make-up bugs

Clean out your make-up bag and wash through all your make-up brushes in a light soapy solution.

Every day we use our make-up brushes and sponges by wiping them over our face and pores. We then return them to the bag and leave them for a further day, slightly damp – perfect conditions for germs to thrive!

A quick shampoo for brushes and sponges will detox your make-up bag!

# Pine

Pine essential oil is refreshing, uplifting and stimulating. It has a boosting effect on the circulation and helps to remove any phlegm or mucus conditions caused by detoxing.

# Be in the moment

A Buddhist philosophy that improves your quality of life immensely.

If you concentrate on what is happening now and what is certain then you deal with things as and when they occur. If you get 'out of the moment' you start to worry about things that may never even happen.

Stay in the moment and detox the long-term worrying from your life.

## Snacks

Snack on dried fruit and nuts rather than crisps and sweets. Feel the energy flow for several hours rather than a quick sugar high and then a lethargic low.

Fruits and nuts are also packed with nutrients and goodness.

# Get a hobby

Stop wasting time and letting it slip away – boredom is exhausting.

Get a hobby and then, when you have a moment, use it to your benefit – you will feel stimulated and challenged. It is much more relaxing to be interested and occupied than bored and restless.

# Detox our ozone

Taking the car is often unavoidable but there are many times when it is *totally* unnecessary.

Do your bit to save the ozone layer and leave the car at home. Take an invigorating walk instead of simply being lazy.

# Ask for help

No man is an island. If you need help then be big enough to ask for it.

If someone asks you for help then you feel flattered that you can make a contribution. It is the same if you ask for help. It means you value your friends' input and their contribution – they will feel flattered too.

Get the job done. Don't struggle when you could do a much better job with just a little help – so just ask for it.

# Kelp

Kelp contains iodine, essential for metabolism, thyroid production, reproduction and growth.

Kelp can be found in seafood, shellfish and seaweed, or can be taken in supplement form.

Boost your circulation and maintain a steady metabolic rate.

## 24-hour fast

After following a mini, mini fast you can
attempt a full, 24-hour fast.

Eat vegetables, fish and rice the day before;
eat nothing for 24 hours but make sure
you drink at least 3 pints of fluid;
then eat vegetables, rice and fish
the day after.

You will emerge feeling lean, clean
and refreshed.
(If you need to nibble then grapes
are allowed!)

# Cut out common irritants

Flour, wheat, caffeine, alcohol, dairy products, sugars, additives and preservatives are all common culprits causing wheezing, allergies, tiredness, erratic mood swings or behaviour or just plain bloating.

Cut them out for a month and then introduce them slowly one at a time after this period. Watch for any reaction and you will be able to find if any of them have been the cause of minor or major irritations.

# Hand reflexology

Look up some key pressure points for
hand reflexology and then use them if you
have any aches and pains or stresses or
strains. No one need ever know that by
simply holding your own hand you are
transforming into a healthy, calm individual.

# Affirmations

Do 5 affirmations a day and talk yourself into anything. Repeat out loud so that you hear them as well as think them.

I deserve health.
I deserve wealth.
I deserve happiness.
I am good at my job.
I have a good life.
My body is healthy.
My mind is wise.

Whatever you want, just say it often enough and you will achieve your dreams.

# Save up for something

Think of something that you would like and have never done or had because you think it is too indulgent, and then save for it.

Use spare change.
Do odd jobs.
Check down the side of the sofa.
Buy budget washing powder.
Walk to work.

It will feel so much better when you have truly earned it – not the least bit indulgent but totally deserved!

# Epsom salts baths every month

Put 2 lbs of Epsom salts into a warm bath.
Relax in the bath for 5 minutes.
Massage your flesh for 5 minutes.
Get out and dry down.
Wrap up warmly for at least an hour.

Feel the toxins purge from your body and feel your body soak up the magnesium for essential use.

Retire relaxed and totally cleansed.

# Grapefruity

Cleanse the air by burning Grapefruit
essential oil.

Grapefruit refreshes and revitalises.

Detox the very air you breathe.

# Invest in a loofah

Exfoliation is the key to skin breathing.

Slough away all dead skin cells to
see your flesh glow and feel your
circulation buzz.

Concentrate on rough spots on the
elbows, feet and knees and slip into a
new day feeling smooth and soft.

# Rice cakes

Munch them to your heart's content.

High in fibre.
Full of roughage.
Tasty.
Low calorie.
Cleansing.
Non-irritant.
Filling.
Crunchy.

The ultimate snack experience.

You could even try the organic chocolate-coated variety for a heavenly munch.

# Home-made hummus

Make the ultimate snack experience even tastier by dipping it into a superb nutritious home-made hummus.

3 oz chick peas
2 oz tahini
Juice of 2 lemons
2 cloves of garlic
2 fl oz olive oil/sunflower oil

Blend together and tuck right in – oil for skin, garlic for circulation and immunity, lemons for cleansing, chick peas for nutrients and energy.

# Dry skin brushing

As well as exfoliation, dry skin brushing is great for sloughing off dead skin cells, kick starting your lymph system and boosting circulation.

Using a soft brush, brush from feet to knees, knees to hips, hands to elbows, elbows to shoulders and round and round your belly.

Feel warm and invigorated.

# Develop your personal 'calm kit'

There is bound to be a quick way to get you into a good mood – you just have to find it. Try the following:

Play music loudly.
Call a friend for a chat.
Take a brisk walk.
Have a bath.
Smell some essential oils.

Find the key to changing your moods and next time you can snap out of it just as soon as you want to!

## Get back to the earth

Do some gardening, get back to the earth
and tend to natural, growing plants.

Turn the soil, weed the weeds and
plant some seeds.

Put something back into Mother Earth
and improve your environment.

## Multivitamin supplements

During the first few weeks of detox you
can supplement your diet with a good
multivitamin. This will provide your body
with the essential vitamins and minerals
during your conversion from bad to good.

## Maintain your metabolic rate

Detox is a programme not a diet.

Make sure that all your internal organs are working and not slowing down by keeping your food intake up. If you feel tired or lethargic you are not eating enough or not eating a good cross section of the food categories: fruit, vegetables, rice, pulses, non-dairy milks and cheeses, oils, fish, herbs and fluids.

The more effectively your organs work the more they can detox.

## Colonic irrigation

If you have ever wondered about c then now is the time to try.

Colonic irrigation will speed up the process and you should feel the k almost immediately.

Find a reputable practitioner and k session – experience something di

# Say 'No!'

Just say 'No'. If someone wants something that you cannot give – energy, time, brain power – or something that would make your personal stocks dangerously low like emotional or physical help, then just say 'No'.

Wait until you feel ready to give freely and then you will be much more helpful without damaging yourself.

You cannot help if you have nothing left to give.

# Try yoga

Yoga can relax, tone and invigorate. You can attend a few classes to learn the basics or get a book that takes you through the elementary steps. Do a short yoga session every day.

Maintaining flexibility will give you a healthier, fitter life.

# Clean your windows

Let the light shine through and the
energy flow freely.
If the windows are dirty then your outlook
on the world is clouded.
If your windows are clean and the light
gets through then your view is crystal clear.

# Potassium

Our bodies need twice as much potassium
as sodium to keep an efficient fluid balance
within the body and prevent
high blood pressure.

It is too easy to have a salt rich diet and
miss out on the potassium. Eat more raw
vegetables, green vegetables, dried fruit
and apricots and keep the balance.

# Fresh fruit to start the day

Start every day with a cleansing and refreshing fresh fruit salad. Make a load at the weekend, store it in an airtight container in the fridge and tuck in every morning.

Nutritious, light and refreshing breakfasts 7 days a week.

# Brown rice

Convert to brown rice – it's scouring and cleansing. It absorbs all the waste in your intestine and flushes it out efficiently.

Short grain is best as it has a larger surface area and can absorb even more. Boil a pan full and have some with each meal.

# Ask for something you want

If you don't ask you don't get.

If you want a promotion – ask for it.
If you want time off – ask for it.
If you want help – ask for it.

Danger – asking for something may result
in you getting it!

# Raw food

Have at least one meal a day consisting of
entirely raw food.

Raw vegetables.
Raw salad.
Oil and lemon juice 'raw' dressing.
NB  You can mix these with boiled
brown rice.

Raw food is raw energy.

# Smile

Smile all day at everything and everyone
that deserves a smile and see how many
smiles you get back.

Detox the gloom and make
the place sunny.

## Pretty in pink

Wear a colour you have never worn before
and see how it makes you feel.

Be bold and put on a splash.

Feel uplifted and interesting.

# Toxins

Take antioxidants and banish the toxins.

# Filter your own water

Get a water filter in your fridge and save money on bottled water. Be sure to renew your filters.

Fresh, clear water 'on tap', to help purify and cleanse your body.

# Be your own best friend

If your best friend has been working hard
or has been through a bad time then you
think of them and decide to give them a
treat to 'take them away from it all'.
Well, now is the time to be your own
best friend.

Decide what you deserve and jolly well go
and do it. It doesn't have to be big but just
something that helps you recognise how
great you are.

# Clear your clutter

Look at your desk/workplace/home – the place where you spend most of your day – and clear anything that you don't need, use or have just let hang around.

In the principles of feng shui if you have a cluttered desk then you cannot think straight – you have a cluttered head.

Detox your workstation and move onwards and upwards.

# Digest properly

Chew your food at least 15 times and savour the flavour. How many times have you got through a meal and really only tasted the first mouthful? If you slow down and chew everything you will actually taste the food and make digestion much, much more efficient.

A double bonus for mind *and* body!

# Digest properly 2

Chew your food properly. It will take you slightly longer to eat your meal, but you will give your stomach time to tell your brain that you are full.

This is likely to result in you eating less as it takes 20 minutes for your brain to register this message – by which time we have normally eaten far too much and feel hugely bloated.

Savour flavour and save calories.

## Detox tiredness

If you get tired or stressed during the
day simply:
Move away from your desk or situation.
Have a long tall stretch.
Bend down to touch the floor.
Twist your body slowly from side to side.
Tense every muscle and then
relax every muscle.
Go all floppy.
Shake yourself down and start afresh.

# Drain your lymph

Book yourself in for a Lymph Drainage Massage and give your body a helping hand to speed up and clear through your own waste disposal system.

If you are feeling a bit sluggish and 'toxed' then this will do the trick.

# Forget bad snacks and go for good snacks

Fill the gap with delicious crudités, dried fruits or nutty nuts and, if you like, rice cakes – munch away to your heart's content.

No additives, preservatives or colourings – just plain hearty food for life.

# Banish stimulants

Cut out caffeine, alcohol, sugar and refined foods.

Cutting these out will eliminate all the highs and lows that we put our body through when including them in our day-to-day diet.

Cut out stimulants and stay balanced and constant.

# Create your own spa at home

Run a bath, light some candles, add some olive oil to the bath water, add some essential oils, cut circles of cucumber for your eyes and mix honey and salt for a facial scrub.

Soak for half an hour and when you get out – slowly as the oil is slippery – pad yourself dry with a towel and rub in the oils as natural moisturiser. Rinse off the face scrub with cool water and go to bed. Awake feeling refreshed and revived.

# Eliminate toxic radiation

Steer clear of any pesticides.
Remove your electric bedside alarm.
Forget the microwave cooking.
Don't sit too close to the TV.

And drastically reduce your exposure
to toxic radiation.

# Mainline Echinacea

Take Echinacea supplements every day and boost your immune system, eliminate colds and flu – even if you have a cold it's not too late to start taking it. Keep yourself looking and feeling younger with its anti-ageing properties and benefit from the antibiotic effects.

All this for just 15 drops, 3 times a day, in water.

# Fake it

Give up sunbathing, you know it's bad for you but you still do it. Now is the time to give up. Cover up in factor 15 or more and just enjoy the warmth and glow it gives everything without burning through your skin and possibly causing cancer.

Apply fake tan if you need to, but a fresh healthy complexion in any colour is better than a wrinkled, walnut one.

# Detox the negative ions

Negative ions cause tiredness and lethargy
and you get them from computer screens,
so make sure you work at least 50 cms
from your screen and take regular breaks.

Make the negative positive!

# Detox even more bad stuff

Get a shield for your mobile phone. The reports are still being written regarding illness resulting from heavy use of mobile phones, so beat the results by investing in a protective case.

Zap the bad vibes not the brain cells.

# Space clearing

Clear the space in your home and revitalise the stale energy. Your home can be invigorated and re-energised with just one morning's 'weird stuff'.

Move all the furniture into the centre of the room. Sprinkle sea salt around the edges, every nook and cranny. Play some loud music or clap your hands whilst walking the perimeter of the room. Then vacuum up all the salt and put the furniture back in the same place or rearrange it.

See how the next few weeks feel more positively charged.

# Make like Tarzan

If you are feeling tired and need a bit more energy then simply thump your own chest like Tarzan and you will feel instantly uplifted.

The area in the centre of your chest just over the sternum will stimulate energy release – yelping like Tarzan helps too!

Ya . . . ahahahaha . . . aaaaaa!

# Keep your complexion young

Using an old toothbrush (softer, bashed down bristles), brush the skin on your face in an upward direction. This will stimulate circulation, slough off dead skin cells, make your face glow and tone your muscles.

It works for superstars so it should work for you.

# Write to yourself

You know how nice it is to receive an unexpected letter telling you some news or just keeping you updated, so drop yourself a line. Tell yourself all your news and everything that is going well in your life.

It's all too easy to let the good bits go unnoticed and unappreciated so get the pen out and hear your own great news.

## Detox speed up

Fennel, Juniper, Geranium

Rub a few drops of one of the above diuretic oils (makes you go to the loo) on the soles of your feet and stimulate the pressure point for the kidneys. Speed up the body's elimination of toxins.

# Change something

Do something differently from now on.

Bath don't shower.
Wear high heels not flatties.
Slice the boiled egg instead of peeling it.
Dry your hair straight don't leave it curly.
Go to bed early not late.

A change is as good as a rest.
And you deserve a rest.

# Tell someone you know how brilliant they are

You know how you think all your friends are brilliant at something or have a real talent – well, next time you see them, tell them.

Even if it's something as simple as they look really good in that top, then just tell them.

It will make you both feel great and it doesn't cost a thing.

# Get rid of bad

Every time something bad happens, take a deep breath and add a comment that makes it OK.

You get cut up in your car – but that's OK because everyone makes mistakes.
You have a bad hair day – but that's OK because you can wear your new hat to cover it up.
You forget to enter the lottery – but that's OK because it means you've won a pound.

# Another reason to eat garlic

It slows down the ageing process.

Raw, tablets, pearls, odourless or not,
there is no end to its benefits – so get
some now.

# You have the time

Saying 'I just don't have the time' becomes a self-fulfilling prophecy. It makes you sound hard done by and that your life is a struggle and you start to believe it.

The truth is that you did have the time but you were doing something else with it.

So if you want to do something, just rearrange and re-prioritise or simply say 'No' to all the things you don't want/need to do. Spend some time living your own life and not everyone else's.

# Go nuts

Nuts are high in nutrients and an excellent source of essential unsaturated fatty acids. They are a rich source of potassium and fibre.

Eat a small handful of raw, unsalted nuts a day and feel the benefits.

# Eat at least 3 meals a day

Another way to keep our metabolic rate from slumping into very low lows and hitting racing highs is to eat regular meals.

Eating 3 meals a day should be an absolute minimum and ideally we should eat 5 smaller meals spread evenly across the day.

This will keep a good balance of energy through the day, keep your mind fresh and alert and give you more time to do the things you want.

# It's all in the timing

Eat your first meal within an hour of getting up and then your last meal at least 4 hours before you go to bed.

This gives you the fuel to start the day and the time your body needs to digest the day.

Be kind to your body and it will be kind to you!

# Find your element and get support from your surroundings

Have a feng shui consultation and find your supportive elements – earth, air, fire, water or metal.

Either buy a book or speak to a specialist and find out how the five elements can support your personal, professional and family life. Work with them to see how much more supported you feel as you go about your daily business.

# Try something for yourself

Don't live your life by other people the whole time. Take some time to try something that might not necessarily please everyone else but would give you great satisfaction – we only get one go at life so why don't we make it a good one.

Better to have had your wish than wish you had.

# Get some therapy

Make some time once a month to have a treatment.

You could have aromatherapy, reflexology, go to a yoga class, book a pedicure or get a facial.

Anything that makes you feel good from the inside and from the outside.

You take your car for a regular service without thinking about it so start to schedule your own ongoing MOT.

# Get some sleep

Sleep keeps us awake and alert, but lack of it can drive us to irrational actions and even madness.

Plan to be in bed before 10.00 p.m. at least one night a week, and asleep by 10.30 p.m.!

Refresh your body and wake up feeling revived and energised.

# Get rid of headaches
# in one easy step

Try any of the following next time you get a headache. Find out which is best for you and learn your key to instant pain relief.

Apply pressure to the top of your big toe – reflexology links the toe with the head. Massage your temples firmly – pressure applied and released will ease tension. Sniff some drops of Lavender essential oil – Lavender will banish headaches in even the most stubborn cases.

# Bach flower remedies

There is a Bach flower remedy for nearly every emotion. If you don't want to find out about all of them then taking their Rescue Remedy will give you relief from many common emotional upsets.

Get some comfort in a bottle – calm is just a few drops away.

# Add a new dimension

Do a course just for the heck of it.

Sign onto something that has vaguely interested you and see how many new horizons it gives you.

New friends, new thoughts, new interests, new stimuli and a fresh outlook.

# Know when to let go

Do you have a friend who always gets you down, points out your shortcomings, only thinks about themselves, takes and never gives – emotionally or physically?

Then decide you don't need them anymore and stop seeing them.

If a relationship is going badly then everyone says it should be 'finished before someone gets hurt'. Well, do the same with a damaging friendship and make more time for your true friends.

# More water

Drink 3 pints or 1.5 litres of filtered or bottled water every day.

No – not *déjà vu* – just more reasons to get you to drink more water.

It wakes you up, gives you more energy, fills you up and gives your body the fluid it needs to operate.

If you get thirsty you are already on your way to dehydration.

# Loosen your belt

We are a belt nation and tend to cut ourselves off at the middle by using belts or tight waistbands. We wear high shoes that put pressure on our legs and take in our jeans to get a more svelte line.

Loosen your belt and increase your circulation.
Free up your internal organs and see how much more relaxed and free you feel.

The very reason Lycra was invented!

# Empty your handbag/briefcase

Take some time to empty and clean out
your handbag or briefcase.

Leave only the essential items, throw out
the rubbish and file what you need.

Remove the excess 'baggage'
from your life.

# Scrape your tongue

Many Eastern cultures scrape the surface of their tongues every morning as they believe this reduces the amount of infections and germs we carry.

Scrape your tongue with your toothbrush and remove all the 'slime' from the day before.

A fresher start to the day.

# Are you totally fulfilled?

List all the roles you play and make sure that they each get equal attention and fulfilment. Become fully rounded instead of overloaded, under appreciated and unfulfilled.

Sarah the wife.
Sarah the mother.
Sarah the accountant.
Sarah the lover.
Sarah the party animal.

# Challenge your brain cells

Do something that uses a part of the brain
that you don't normally use.

Do maths without a calculator.
See a foreign film and don't look at
the subtitles.
Read a factual book.
Install something using the
instruction manual.

Stimulate your brain and feel inspired.

# Don't cross your legs

Restricting circulation around the hip and thigh area can impede blood flow and increase the effects of cellulite!

Let the blood flow freely and sit with your legs together.

Good circulation helps you to stay healthy and energised.

# Grill, flash fry, steam or eat raw

Look at your cooking techniques and change the unhealthy ones for a more healthy alternative.

Grilling, flash frying, steaming or eating raw food provides more flavour, more texture, more energy and retains more goodness.

(Bad = deep fat fry, microwave, put in a sauce, stews, boiled until soggy.)

# Do something unexpected

Get the kids to cook their supper.
Take your partner out to dinner.
Turn up unannounced with flowers.
Call a long lost friend.
Tell someone you love them.

Spread a little happiness and
feel good yourself.

# Don't beat yourself up about bad habits

Rather than feeling guilty about liking some things that are bad for you, identify them in a list and then allow yourself one bad thing a week.

If you like bacon sandwiches then rather than sneaking them in and feeling so bad you don't actually enjoy them – actively decide you will have one a week. Then you can safely be healthy for the rest of the time and totally enjoy your treat – without any guilt.

# Financial detox

Balance your cheque book.
Save your small change.
Recover all monies owed.

If you keep an eye on your cash flow you
can save any unnecessary charges by
warding off overdrafts, spending when you
have the funds and making the most of
what you have got.

## A new start to the day

Swap the side of the bed you sleep on
or move your bed to a different position.

Start the day with a totally new
perspective and see how it
changes your life.

# Meditate to alleviate

Try meditation and create your own oasis of calm.

Find a quiet, warm room.
Sit comfortably or lie on your back
with legs supported.
Breathe deeply.
Let the thoughts flow through your mind,
don't dwell on anything just let them pass.
As you relax more deeply, clear your head
and focus on the gentle rise and fall of
your breathing.

Spend 5 minutes a day meditating and
emerge totally centred.

# Plan for your future

Write down your future plans, what you really want in life. Put them away and review them every now and then. Are you on track?

Use them to help with decisions – will doing something help fulfil your plans? If 'yes' do it and if 'no' then don't.

Know your destination and you can plan your journey easily and simply. Diversions are fine – then just get back on track.

# Read a book and escape

Choose a book and read it . . .

In bed at night for a few minutes.
On the bus on the way to work.
Whilst waiting in a queue.
During your kids' swimming lessons.

When you are reading it is very hard to think of anything else other than what you are reading about so it offers total escape.

## Sauna/Steam

Treat yourself to saunas and steam treatments.

Sweating out toxins through steam and sauna helps your body eliminate unwanted waste and fluids.

Visit your leisure centre and for a small price get clean on the inside and outside too!

# Indulge yourself

Go on, do it, split rivet, go bananas, do your thing, what the heck, who gives a damn, I'm in charge and I'm here!

Put yourself first every now and then and get the feel good factor – forget what *they* want and do what *you* want.

# Write lists

The shopping list and the 'To Do' list are actually magnificent tools for productivity.

Make lists and cross out each task or purchase until the list has been completed.

Don't forget how much you actually get done in a day and don't forget what you actually need to do in a day. There is nothing more detoxing than watching your chores get completed and 'ticked off'.

## Get friends round
## for the evening

Invite friends around for an impromptu
evening and have some more fun.
It doesn't need to cost much. Ask
everyone to bring something to eat
and something to drink.

Better you all staying in together
than all staying in alone.

# Walk

Down tools and go for a walk.

Put this book down now and go for a wander, just for 5 minutes. Have a stroll and look around you to see what life is doing right now.

It is really easy to focus on yourself and what you are doing all the time, so remember to look around and go for a refreshing walk to clear your mind.

# Get your hair cut

Every time we go through a big life change we go and get a haircut – it signifies a new beginning.

So give yourself a fresh start and get your hair re-styled. The new you can face the future with a totally new outlook.

# And finally ...

What goes around comes around.

If you are positive and give out positive energy you will remain positive.

What you give, you get.

Give your body and mind a totally detoxifying experience and you will reap the benefits for many years to come.

# Other books by Jane Scrivner

*Detox Yourself*

*Detox Your Mind*

*Detox Your Life*
(January 2000)